Human Dental Anatomy

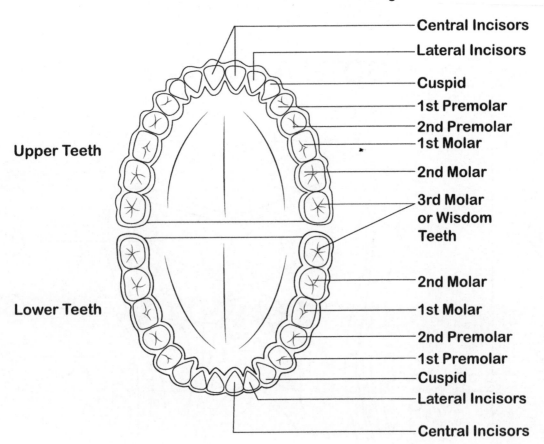

Central Incisors
Lateral Incisors
Cuspid
1st Premolar
2nd Premolar
1st Molar
2nd Molar
3rd Molar or Wisdom Teeth

Upper Teeth

2nd Molar
1st Molar
2nd Premolar
1st Premolar
Cuspid
Lateral Incisors
Central Incisors

Lower Teeth

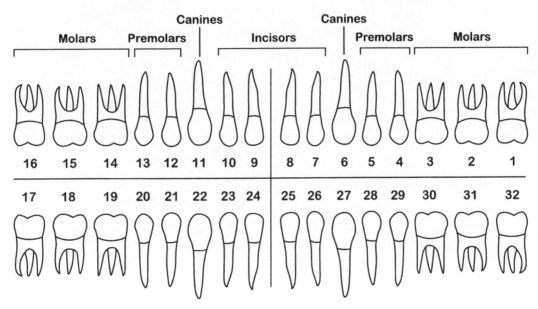

Upper Left   Upper Right

Canines   Canines

Molars   Premolars   Incisors   Premolars   Molars

| 16 | 15 | 14 | 13 | 12 | 11 | 10 | 9 | 8 | 7 | 6 | 5 | 4 | 3 | 2 | 1 |

| 17 | 18 | 19 | 20 | 21 | 22 | 23 | 24 | 25 | 26 | 27 | 28 | 29 | 30 | 31 | 32 |

Lower Left   Lower Right

TOOTH ANATOMY

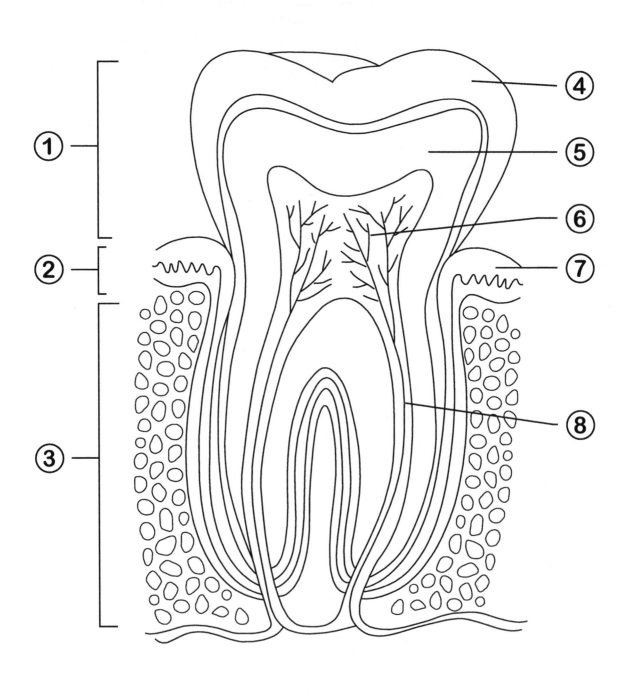

TOOTH ANATOMY

(1). **Crown**

(2). **Neck**

(3). **Root**

(4). **Enamel**

(5). **Dentin**

(6). **Pulp Cavity**

(7). **Gingiva**

(8). **Root Canal**

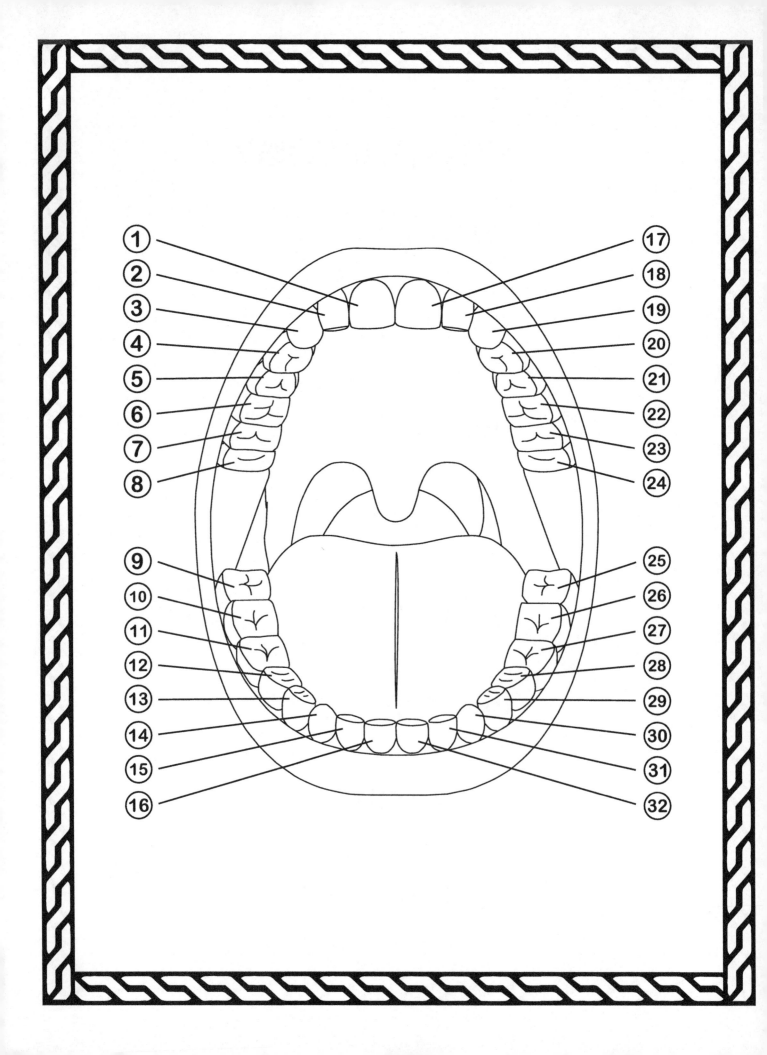

(1). Central Incisor	(17). Central Incisor
(2). Lateral Incisor	(18). Lateral Incisor
(3). Canine	(19). Canine
(4). First Premolar	(20). First Premolar
(5). Second Premolar	(21). Second Premolar
(6). First Molar	(22). First Molar
(7). Second Molar	(23). Second Molar
(8). Third Molar	(24). Third Molar
(9). Third Molar	(25). Third Molar
(10). Second Molar	(26). Second Molar
(11). First Molar	(27). First Molar
(12). Second Premolar	(28). Second Premolar
(13). First Premolar	(29). First Premolar
(14). Canine	(30). Canine
(15). Lateral Incisor	(31). Lateral Incisor
(16). Central Incisor	(32). Central Incisor

TOOTH ANATOMY

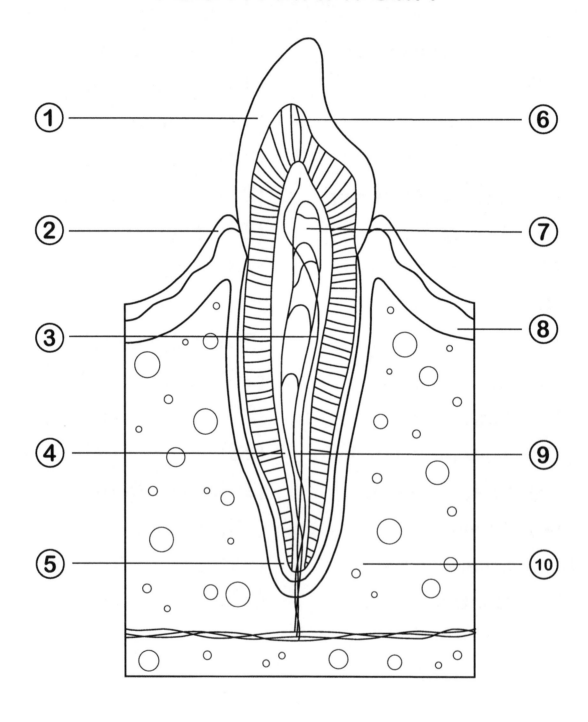

TOOTH ANATOMY

(1). Enamel

(2). Gingiva

(3). Nerve

(4). Root Canal

(5). Cementum

(6). Dentin

(7). Pulp Cavity

(8). Gum Tissue

(9). Blood Vessels

(10). Bone

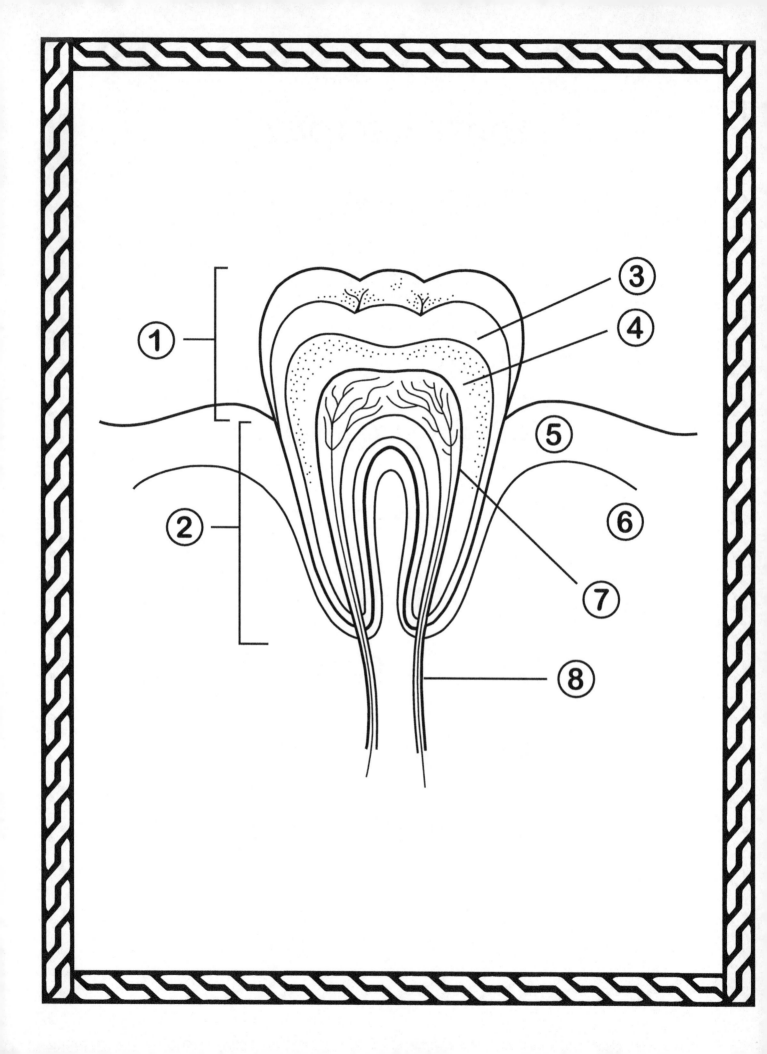

(1). Crown

(2). Root

(3). Enamel

(4). Dentine

(5). Gum

(6). Jaw Bone

(7). Pulp

(8). Nerves and Blood Vessels

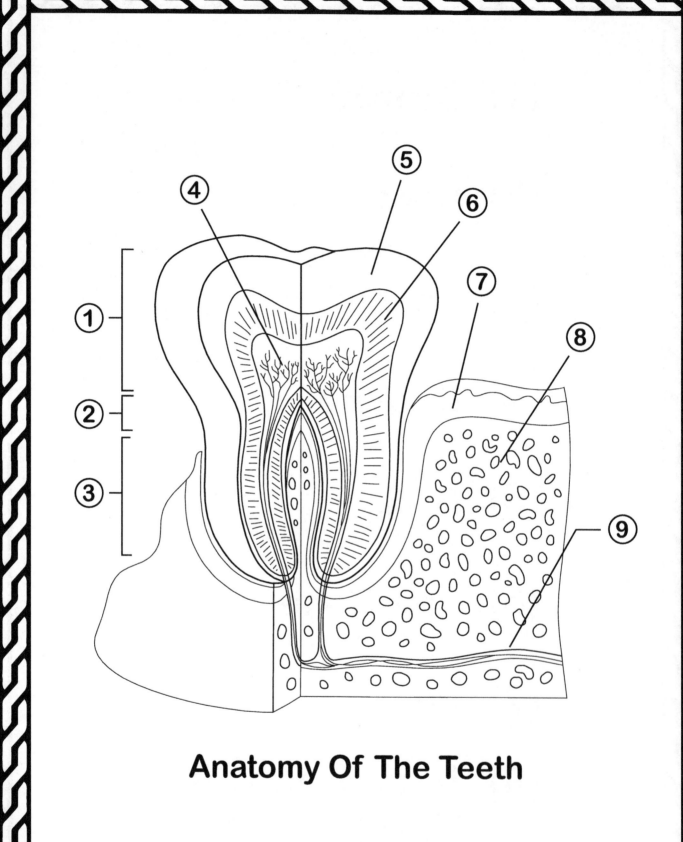

Anatomy Of The Teeth

(1). Crown

(2). Neck

(3). Root

(4). Pulp

(5). Enamel

(6). Dentine

(7). Gum

(8). Jaw Bone

(9). Root Canal

Anatomy Of The Teeth

Milk Tooth / Baby Tooth

Primary Teeth Eruption (Month)

Loss of Deciduous Teeth (Year)

1
2
3
4
5
6
7
8
9
10

11
12
13
14
15
16
17
18
19
20

Milk Tooth / Baby Tooth

Primary Teeth Eruption (Month)

(1). Central incisor (8-12)

(2). Lateral incisor (9-13)

(3). Canine (16-22)

(4). First Molar (13-19)

(5). Second Molar (25-33)

(6). Second Molar (23-31)

(7). First Molar (14-18)

(8). Canine (17-23)

(9). Lateral Incisor (10-16)

(10). Central Incisor (6-10)

Loss of Deciduous Teeth (Year)

(11). Central Incisor (6-7)

(12). Lateral Incisor (7-8)

(13). Canine (10-12)

(14). First Molar (9-11)

(15). Second Molar (10-12)

(16). Second Molar (10-12)

(17). First Molar (9-11)

(18). Canine (9-12)

(19). Lateral Incisor (7-8)

(20). Central Incisor (6-7)

Children Dental Chart

Primary Teeth Eruption (Month)   **Loss of Deciduous Teeth (Year)**

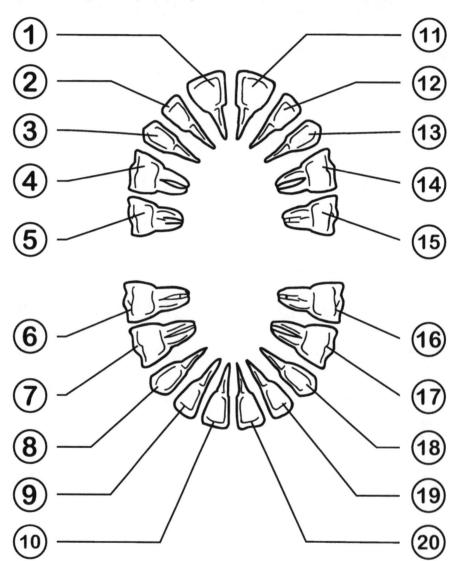

Children Dental Chart

Primary Teeth Eruption (Month)

(1). Central incisor (8-12)

(2). Lateral incisor (9-13)

(3). Canine (16-22)

(4). First Molar (13-19)

(5). Second Molar (25-33)

(6). Second Molar (23-31)

(7). First Molar (14-18)

(8). Canine (17-23)

(9). Lateral incisor (10-16)

(10). Central incisor (6-10)

Loss of Deciduous Teeth (Year)

(11). Central incisor (6-7)

(12). Lateral incisor (7-8)

(13). Canine (10-12)

(14). First Molar (9-11)

(15). Second Molar (10-12)

(16). Second Molar (10-12)

(17). First Molar (9-11)

(18). Canine (9-12)

(19). Lateral incisor (7-8)

(20). Central incisor (6-7)

Tooth Chart

Primary Teeth (Upper Teeth)

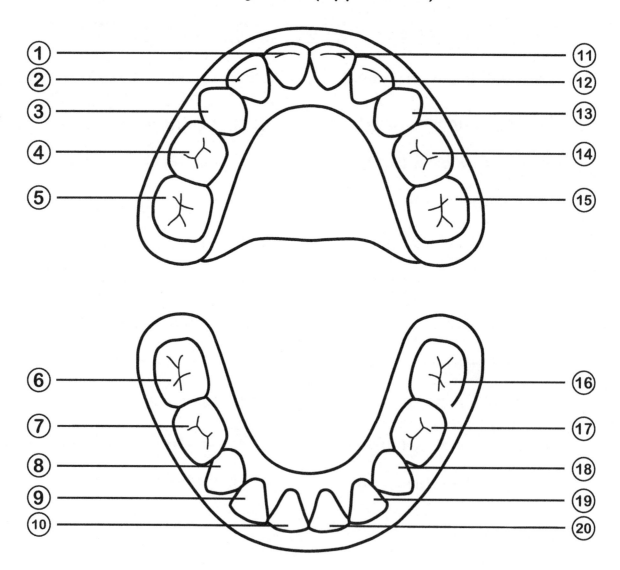

Primary Teeth (Lower Teeth)

Tooth Chart

Primary Teeth (Upper Teeth)

(1). Central Incisor

(2). Lateral Incisor

(3). Canine (Cuspid)

(4). First Molar

(5). Second Molar

(6). Second Molar

(7). First Molar

(8). Canine (Cuspid)

(9). Lateral Incisor

(10). Central Incisor

(11). Central Incisor

(12). Lateral Incisor

(13). Canine (Cuspid)

(14). First Molar

(15). Second Molar

(16). Second Molar

(17). First Molar

(18). Canine (Cuspid)

(19). Lateral Incisor

(20). Central Incisor

Primary Teeth (Lower Teeth)

Eruption

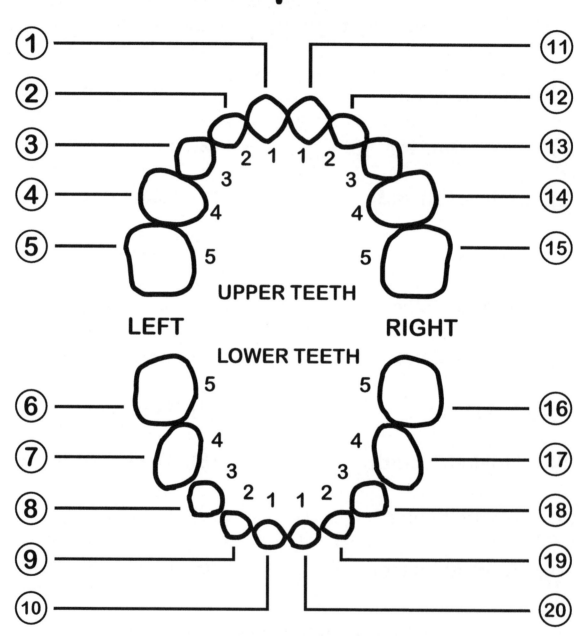

UPPER TEETH

LEFT · RIGHT

LOWER TEETH

Eruption

(1). 8-12 Months

(2). 9-13 Months

(3). 16-23 Months

(4). 13-19 Months

(5). 23-23 Months

(6). 23-31 Months

(7). 14-18 Months

(8). 17-23 Months

(9). 10-16 Months

(10). 6-10 Months

(11). Central Incisor

(12). Lateral Incisor

(13). Canine (Cuspid)

(14). First Molar

(15). Second Molar

(16). Second Molar

(17). First Molar

(18). Canine (Cuspid)

(19). Lateral Incisor

(20). Central Incisor

Shedding

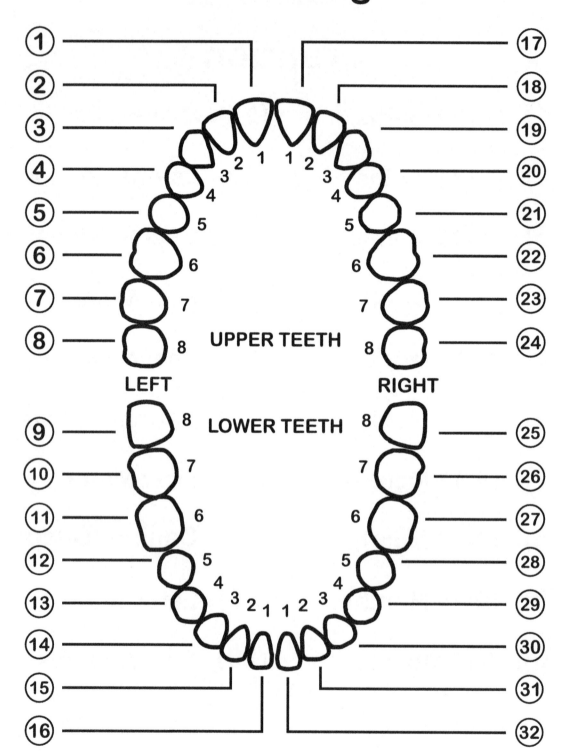

UPPER TEETH

LEFT RIGHT

LOWER TEETH

Shedding

(1). 7-8 Years

(2). 8-9 Years

(3). 11-12 Years

(4). 10-11 Years

(5). 10-12 Years

(6). 6-7 Years

(7). 11-13 Years

(8). 17-21 Years

(9). 17-21 Years

(10). 11-13 Years

(11). 6-7 Years

(12). 11-12 Years

(13). 10-12 Years

(14). 9-10 Years

(15). 7-8 Years

(16). 6-7 Years

(17). Central Incisor

(18). Lateral Incisor

(19). Canine (Cuspid)

(20). First Premolar

(21). Second Premolar

(22). First Molar

(23). Second Molar

(24). Third Molar

(25). Third Molar

(26). Second Molar

(27). First Molar

(28). Second Premolar

(29). First Premolar

(30). Canine (Cuspid)

(31). Lateral Incisor

(32). Central Incisor

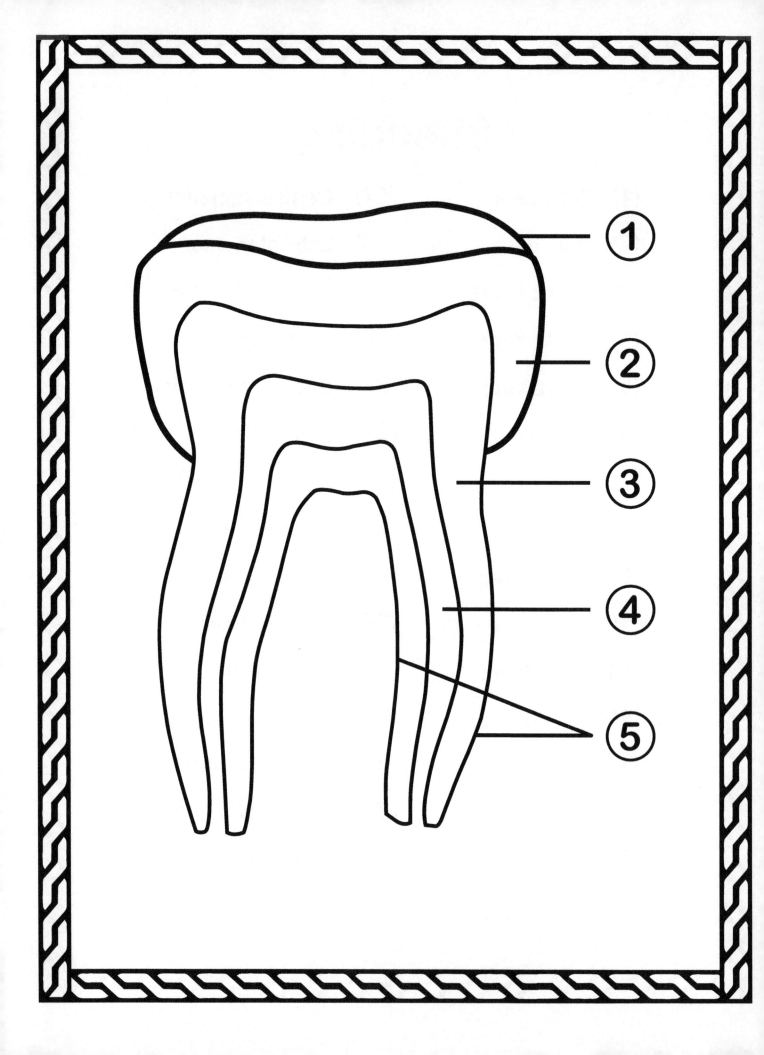

(1). Pellicle

(2). Enamel

(3). Dentin

(4). Pulp

(5). Cementum

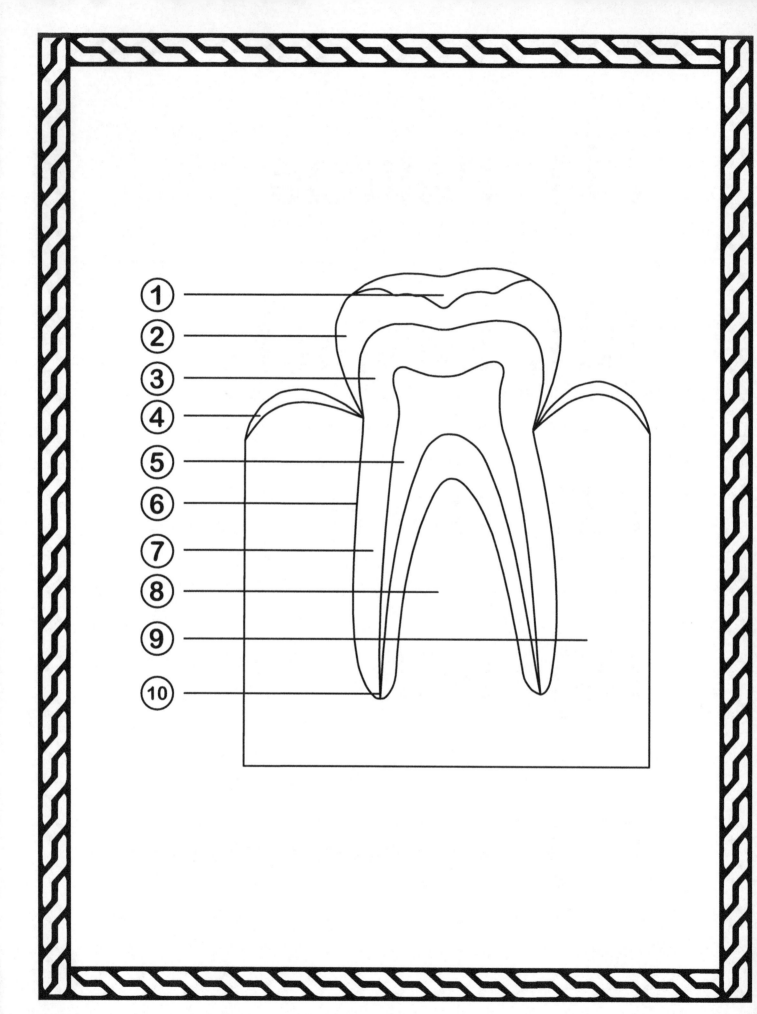

(1). Fissure

(2). Enamel

(3). Dentine

(4). Gum

(5). Pulp

(6). Periodont

(7). Cement Root

(8). Jawbone

(9). Bone

(10). Apical Aperture

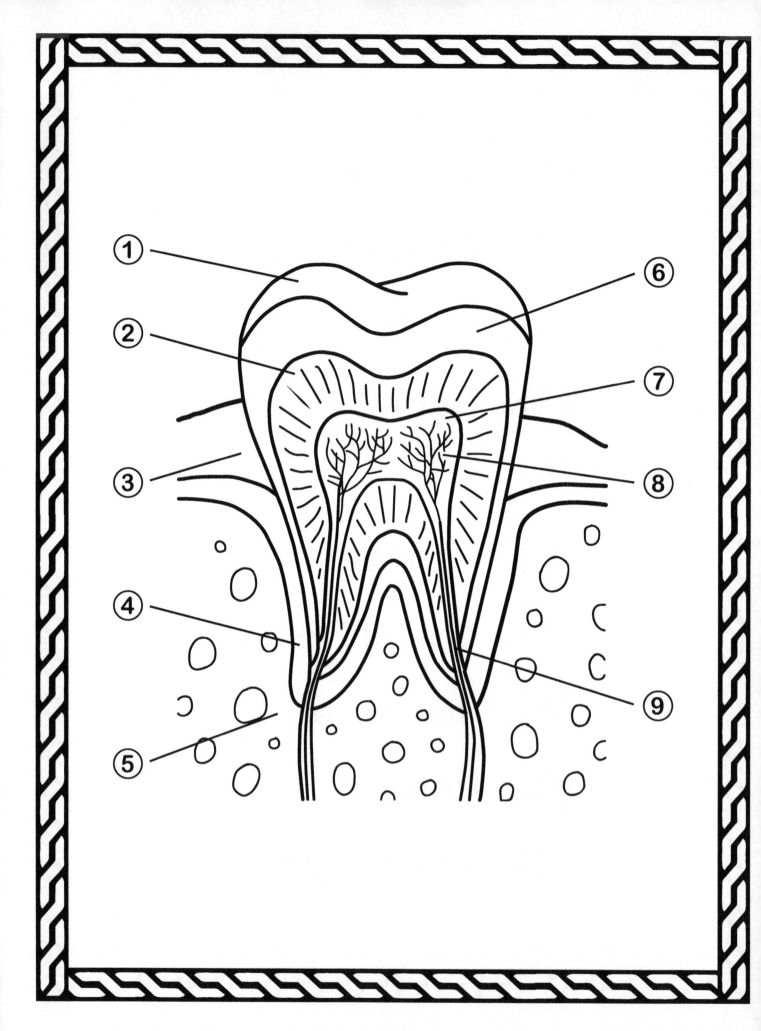

(1). Cusp

(2). Dentin

(3). Gingiva

(4). Periodontal Fibre

(5). Jaw Bone

(6). Enamel

(7). Pulp Cavity

(8). Nerves

(9). Blood Vessels

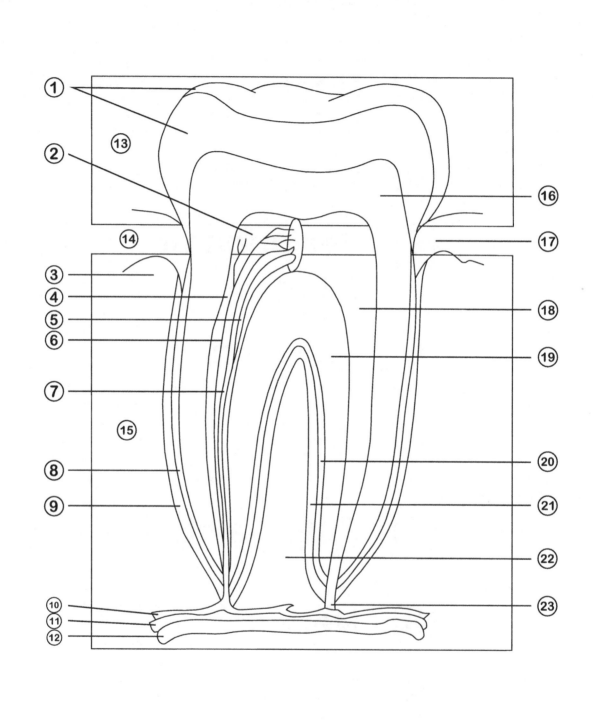

(1). Enamel

(2). Pulp Cavity

(3). Alveolar Bone

(4). Root Canal

(5). Vein

(6). Nerve

(7). Artery

(8). Cementum

(9). Periodontal Membrane

(10). Nerve

(11). Artery

(12). Vein

(13). Crown

(14). Neck

(15). Root

(16). Dentin

(17). Gingiva

(18). Pulp

(19). Dentin

(20). Cementum

(21). Periodontal Membrane

(22). Alveolar Bone

(23). Root Foramen

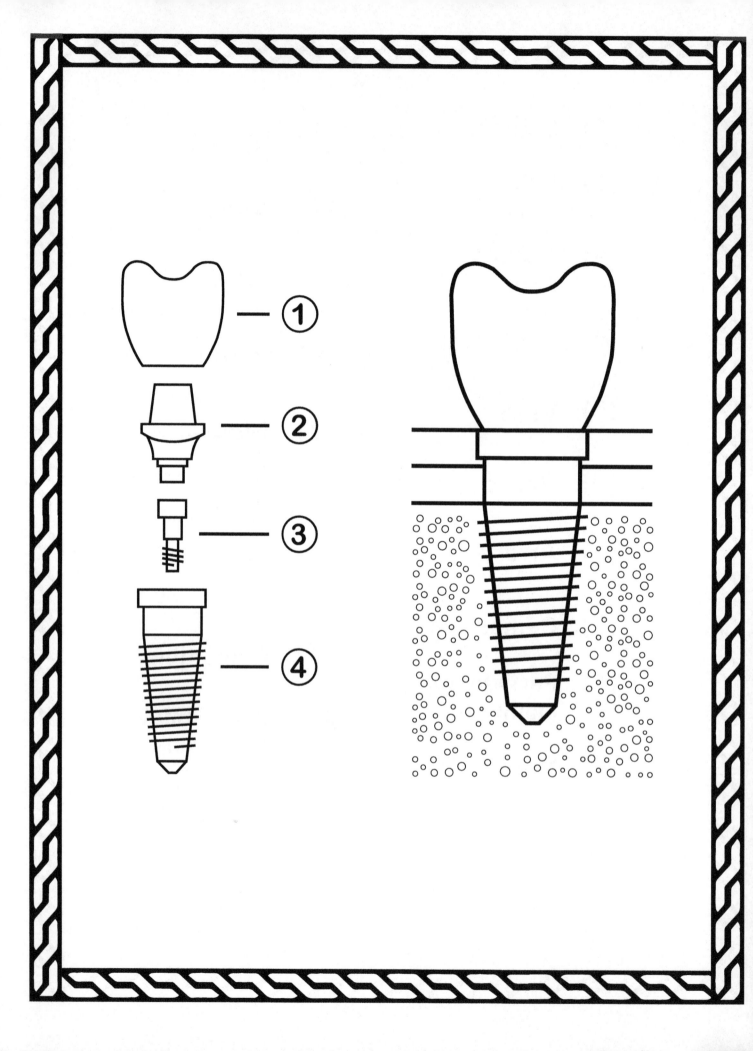

(1). Crown

(2). Abutment

(3). Screw

(4). Implant

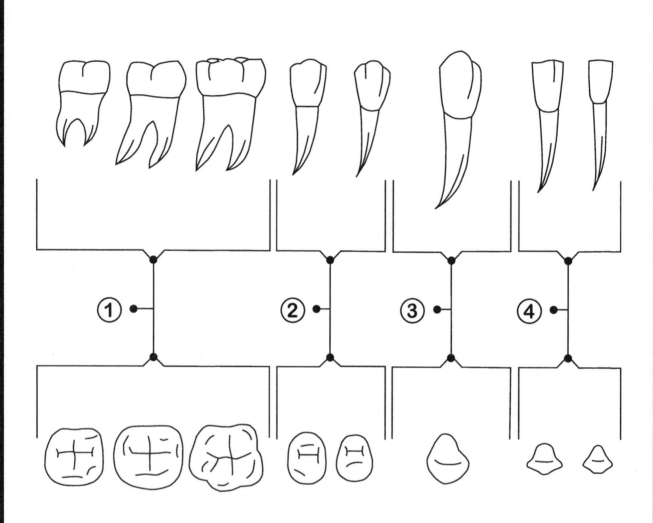

LOWER JAW TEETH

(1). Molars

(2). Premolars

(3). Canines

(4). Incisors

LOWER JAW TEETH

Upper and Lower Teeth

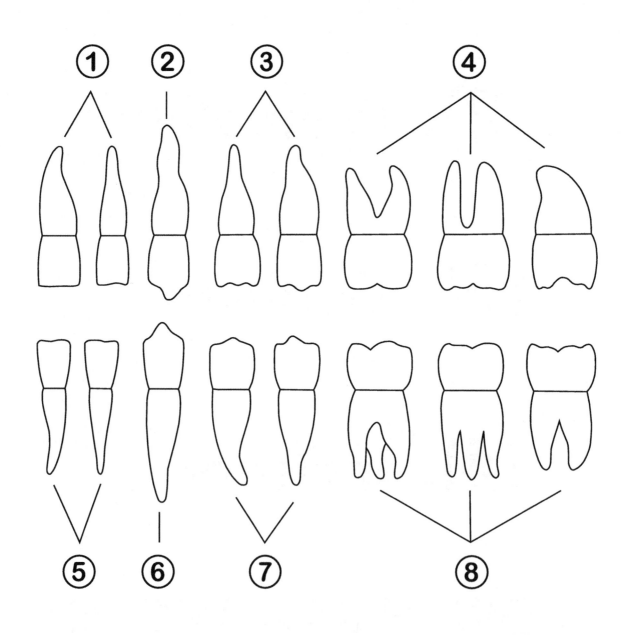

Upper and Lower Teeth

(1). Incisors

(2). Canine

(3). Premolars

(4). Molars

(5). Incisors

(6). Canine

(7). Premolars

(8). Molars

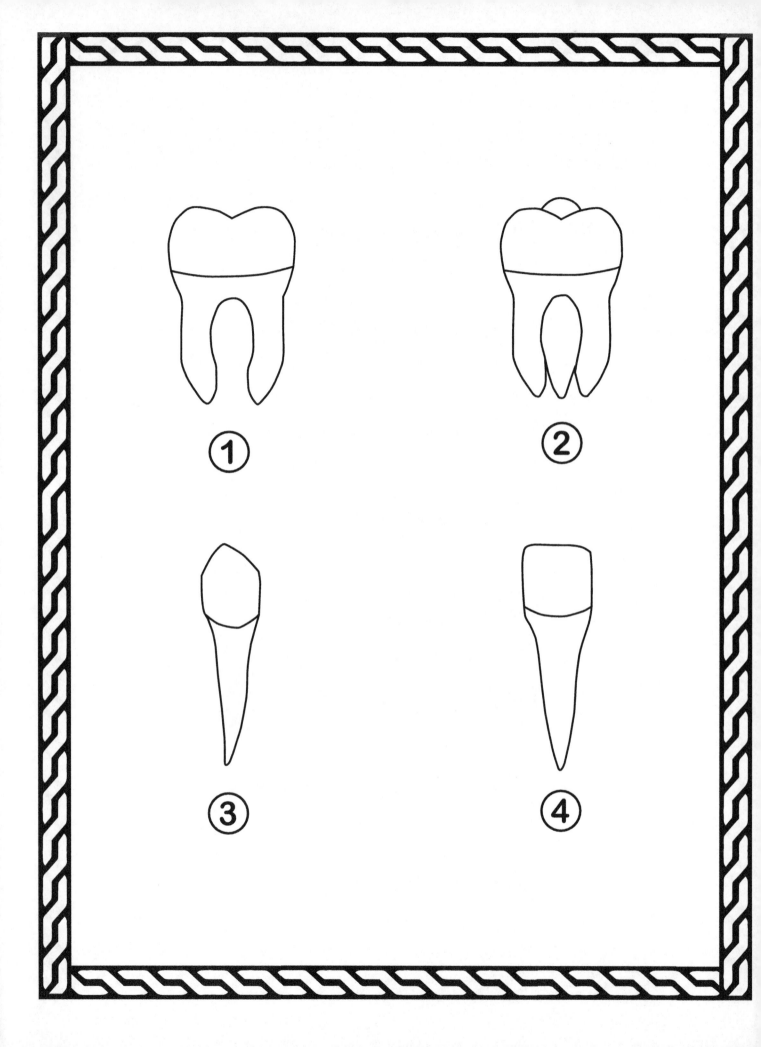

(1). Premolars

(2). Molars

(3). Canines

(4). Incisors

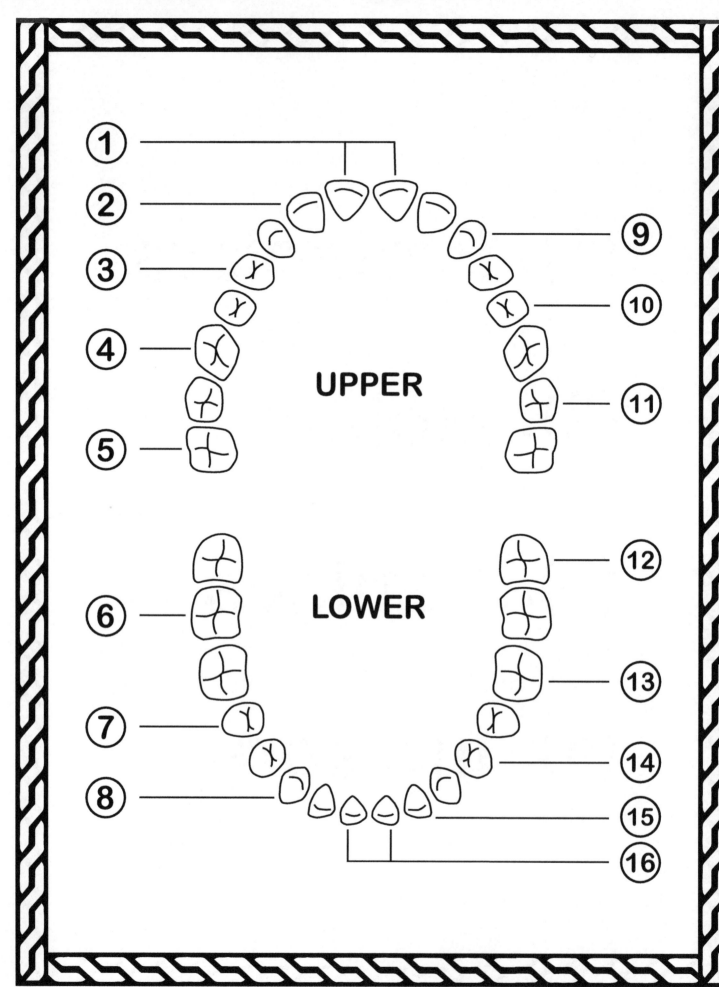

UPPER

LOWER

(1). Central Incisors

(2). Lateral Incisors

(3). First Premolars

(4). First Molars

(5). Third Molars

(6). Second Molars

(7). Second Premolars

(8). Canines / Cuspids

(9). Canines / Cuspids

(10). Second Premolars

(11). Second Molars

(12). Third Molars

(13). First Molars

(14). First Premolars

(15). Lateral Incisors

(16). Central Incisors

Teeth

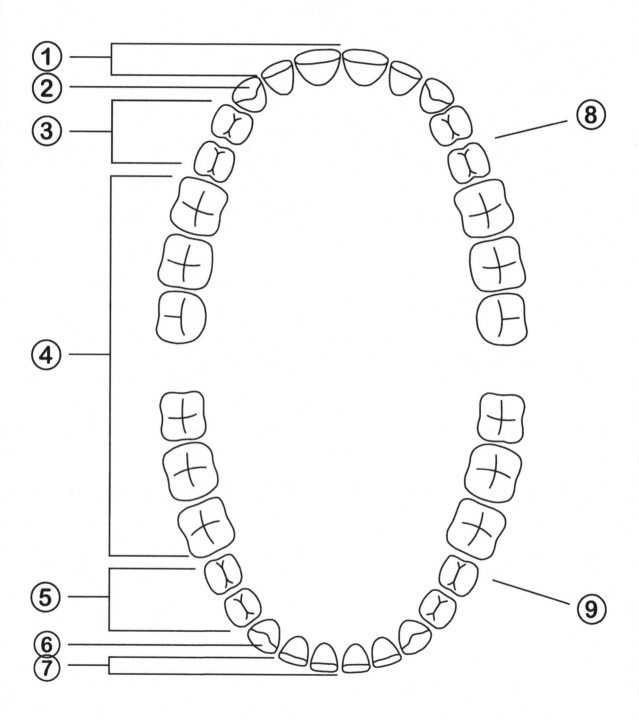

Teeth

(1). Incisors

(2). Canine

(3). Premolars

(4). Molars

(5). Premolars

(6). Canine

(7). Incisors

(8). Upper

(9). Lower

Primary and Secondary teeth

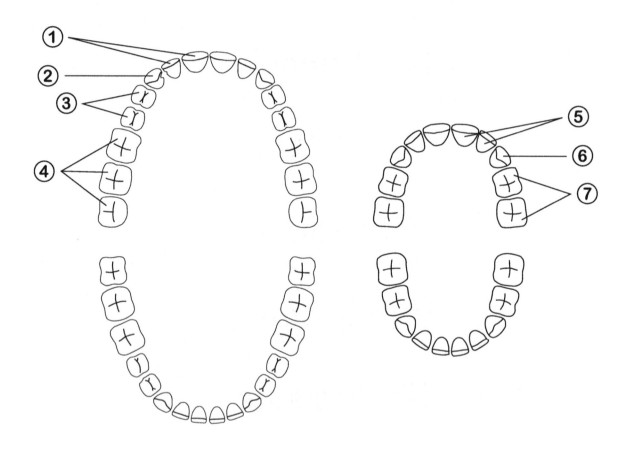

Primary and Secondary teeth

(1). Incisors

(2). Canine

(3). Premolars

(4). Molars

(5). Incisors

(6). Canine

(7). Molars

Milk Teeth

Permanent Teeth

Upper Jaw Teeth

Upper Jaw Teeth

① ——————
② ——————
③ ——————

④ ——————
⑤ ——————

—————— ⑪
—————— ⑫
—————— ⑬
—————— ⑭
—————— ⑮
—————— ⑯
—————— ⑰
—————— ⑱

Lower Jaw Teeth

Lower Jaw Teeth

⑥ ——————
⑦ ——————

⑧ ——————
⑨ ——————
⑩ ——————

—————— ⑲
—————— ⑳
—————— ㉑
—————— ㉒
—————— ㉓
—————— ㉔
—————— ㉕
—————— ㉖

Milk Teeth

Upper Jaw Teeth

(1). 8-12 Months

(2). 9-13 Months

(3). 16-22 Months

(4). 13-19 Months

(5). 25-33 Months

Lower Jaw Teeth

(6). 23-31 Months

(7). 14-18 Months

(8). 17-23 Months

(9). 10-16 Months

(10). 6-10 Months

Permanent Teeth

Upper Jaw Teeth

(11). 7-8 Years

(12). 8-9 Years

(13). 11-12 Years

(14). 10-11 Years

(15). 10-12 Years

(16). 6-7 Years

(17). 12-13 Years

(18). 17-21 Years

Lower Jaw Teeth

(19). 17-21 Years

(20). 11-13 Years

(21). 6-7 Years

(22). 11-12 Years

(23). 10-12 Years

(24). 9-10 Years

(25). 7-8 Years

(26). 6-7 Years

Anatomy of Teeth

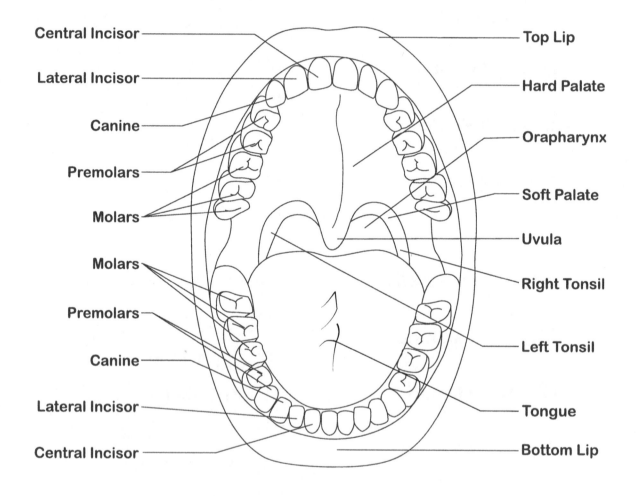

Milk Teeth - Adult Teeth

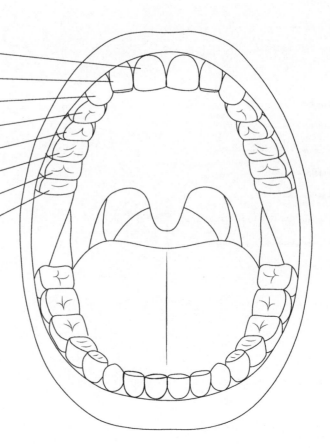

4 Central Incisors
4 Lateral Incisors
4 Canines
4 First Molars
4 Second Molars

20 Milk Teeth

4 Central Incisors
4 Lateral Incisors
4 Canines
4 First Premolars
4 Second Premolars
4 First Molars
4 Second Molars
4 Third Molars

32 Adult Teeth

Permanent and Primary Teeth

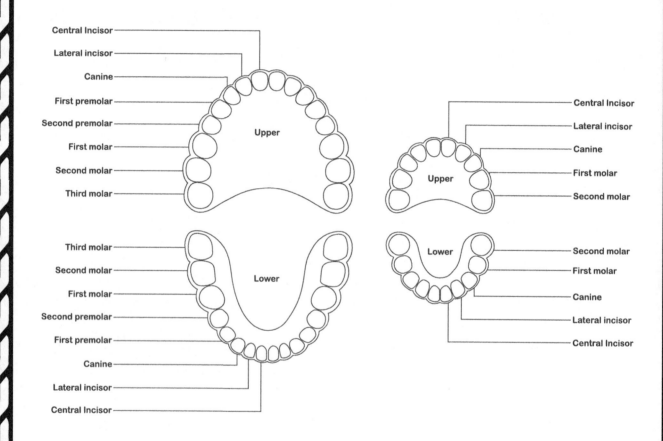

Central Incisor
Lateral incisor
Canine
First premolar
Second premolar
First molar
Second molar
Third molar

Upper

Third molar
Second molar
First molar
Second premolar
First premolar
Canine
Lateral incisor
Central Incisor

Lower

Central Incisor
Lateral incisor
Canine
First molar
Second molar

Upper

Second molar
First molar
Canine
Lateral incisor
Central Incisor

Lower

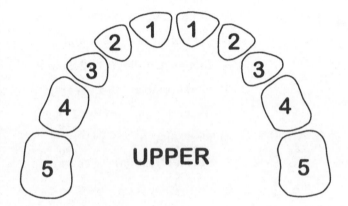

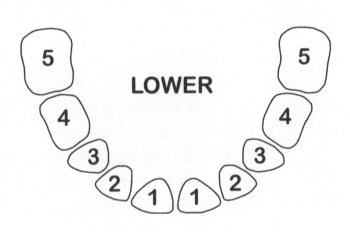

UPPER

1 Central Incisor (8-12 Months)

2 Lateral Incisor (9-13 Months)

3 Canine (Cuspid) (16-22 Months)

4 First Molar (13-19 Months)

5 Second Molar (25-33 Months)

LOWER

1 Central Incisor (6-10 Months)

2 Lateral Incisor (10-16 Months)

3 Canine (Cuspid) (17-23 Months)

4 First Molar (14-18 Months)

5 Second Molar (23-31 Months)

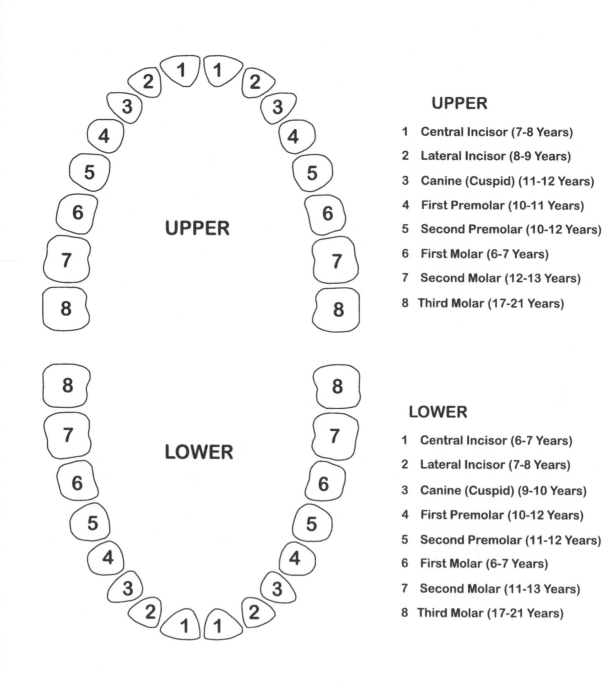

UPPER

1 Central Incisor (7-8 Years)

2 Lateral Incisor (8-9 Years)

3 Canine (Cuspid) (11-12 Years)

4 First Premolar (10-11 Years)

5 Second Premolar (10-12 Years)

6 First Molar (6-7 Years)

7 Second Molar (12-13 Years)

8 Third Molar (17-21 Years)

LOWER

1 Central Incisor (6-7 Years)

2 Lateral Incisor (7-8 Years)

3 Canine (Cuspid) (9-10 Years)

4 First Premolar (10-12 Years)

5 Second Premolar (11-12 Years)

6 First Molar (6-7 Years)

7 Second Molar (11-13 Years)

8 Third Molar (17-21 Years)

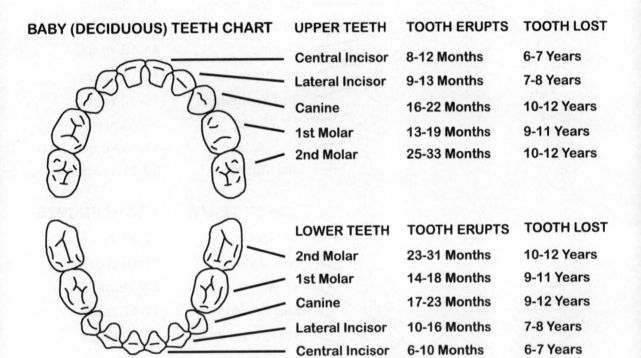

BABY (DECIDUOUS) TEETH CHART

UPPER TEETH	TOOTH ERUPTS	TOOTH LOST
Central Incisor	8-12 Months	6-7 Years
Lateral Incisor	9-13 Months	7-8 Years
Canine	16-22 Months	10-12 Years
1st Molar	13-19 Months	9-11 Years
2nd Molar	25-33 Months	10-12 Years

LOWER TEETH	TOOTH ERUPTS	TOOTH LOST
2nd Molar	23-31 Months	10-12 Years
1st Molar	14-18 Months	9-11 Years
Canine	17-23 Months	9-12 Years
Lateral Incisor	10-16 Months	7-8 Years
Central Incisor	6-10 Months	6-7 Years

ADULT (PERMANENT) TEETH CHART

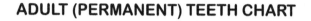

UPPER TEETH	TOOTH ERUPTS
Central Incisor	7-8 Years
Lateral Incisor	8-9 Years
Canine	11-12 Years
1st Premolar	10-11 Years
2nd Premolar	10-12 Years
1st Molar	6-7 Years
2nd Molar	12-13 Years
3rd Molar	17-21 Years

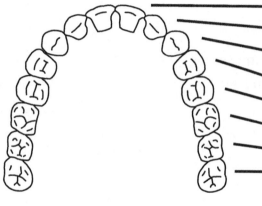

LOWER TEETH	TOOTH ERUPTS
3rd Molar	17-21 Years
2nd Molar	11-13 Years
1st Molar	6-7 Years
2nd Premolar	11-12 Years
1st Premolar	10-12 Years
Canine	9-10 Years
Lateral incisor	7-8 Years
Central incisor	6-7 Years

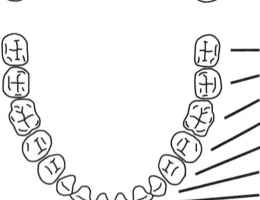

Tooth Chart

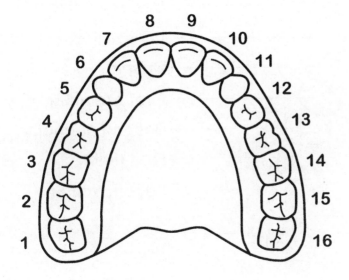

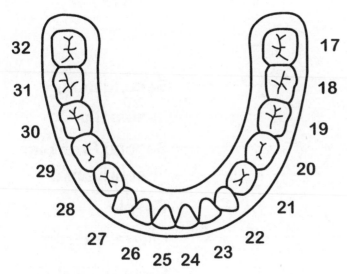

1. 3rd Molar (Wisdom Tooth)
2. 2nd Molar (12-yr Molar)
3. 1st Molar (6-yr Molar)
4. 2nd Bicuspid (2nd Premolar)
5. 1st Bicuspid (1st Premolar)
6. Cuspid (Canine/Eye Tooth)
7. Lateral Incisor
8. Central Incisor
9. Central Incisor
10. Lateral Incisor
11. Cuspid (Canine/Eye Tooth)
12. 1st Bicuspid (1st Premolar)
13. 2nd Bicuspid (2nd Premolar)
14. 1st Molar (6-yr Molar)
15. 2nd Molar (12-yr Molar)
16. 3rd Molar (Wisdom Tooth)
17. 3rd Molar (Wisdom Tooth)
18. 2nd Molar (12-yr Molar)
19. 1st Molar (6-yr Molar)
20. 2nd Bicuspid (2nd Premolar)
21. 1st Bicuspid (1st Premolar)
22. Cuspid (Canine/Eye Tooth)
23. Lateral Incisor
24. Central Incisor
25. Central Incisor
26. Lateral Incisor
27. Cuspid (Canine/Eye Tooth)
28. 1st Bicuspid (1st Premolar)
29. 2nd Bicuspid (2nd Premolar)
30. 1st Molar (6-yr Molar)
31. 2nd Molar (12-yr Molar)
32. 3rd Molar (Wisdom Tooth)

Tooth Anatomy

Upper teeth

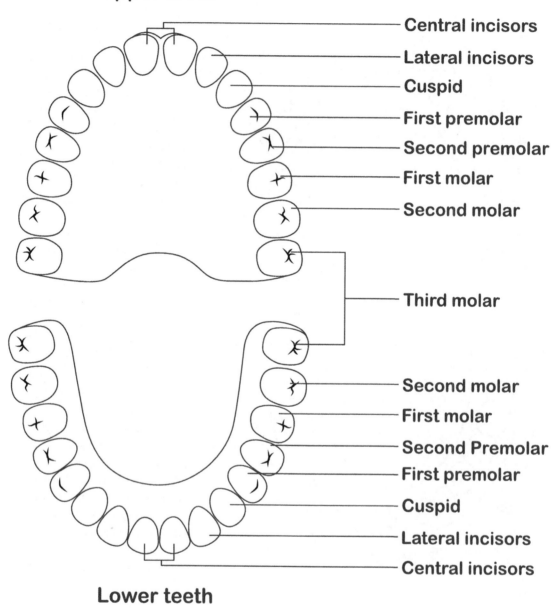

- Central incisors
- Lateral incisors
- Cuspid
- First premolar
- Second premolar
- First molar
- Second molar

- Third molar

- Second molar
- First molar
- Second Premolar
- First premolar
- Cuspid
- Lateral incisors
- Central incisors

Lower teeth

Adult Dental Chart

Eruption (year)

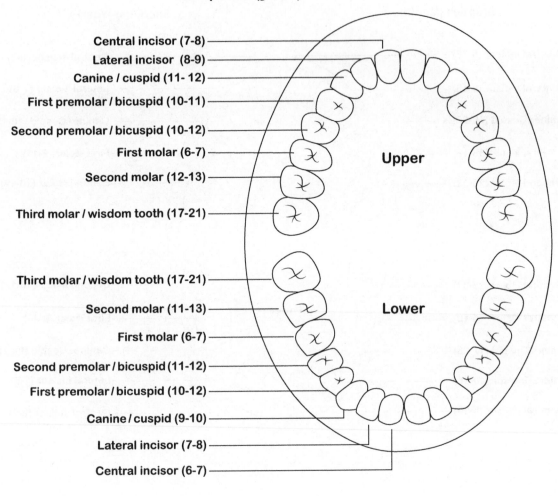

Central incisor (7-8)
Lateral incisor (8-9)
Canine / cuspid (11- 12)
First premolar / bicuspid (10-11)
Second premolar / bicuspid (10-12)
First molar (6-7)
Second molar (12-13)
Third molar / wisdom tooth (17-21)

Upper

Third molar / wisdom tooth (17-21)
Second molar (11-13)
First molar (6-7)
Second premolar / bicuspid (11-12)
First premolar / bicuspid (10-12)
Canine / cuspid (9-10)
Lateral incisor (7-8)
Central incisor (6-7)

Lower

Children Dental Chart

Eruption (Month)   **Shedding (Year)**

Central incisor (8-12) ——————————————————— Central incisor (6-7)

Lateral incisor (9-13) ——————————————————— Lateral incisor (7-8)

Canine / Cuspid (16-22) ——————————————————— Canine / Cuspid (10-12)

First Molar (13-19) ——————————————————— First Molar (9-11)

Second Molar (25-33) ——————————————————— Second Molar (10-12)

Upper

Lower

Second Molar (23-31) ——————————————————— Second Molar (10-12)

First Molar (14-18) ——————————————————— First Molar (9-11)

Canine / Cuspid (17-23) ——————————————————— Canine / Cuspid (9-12)

Lateral incisor (10-16) ——————————————————— Lateral incisor (7-8)

Central incisor (6-10) ——————————————————— Central incisor (6-7)

Adult Dental Anatomy

Upper right:

1. 3rd molar / wisdom tooth
2. 2nd molar
3. 1st molar
4. 2nd premolar
5. 1st premolar
6. Cuspid
7. Lateral incisors
8. Central incisors

Upper left:

9. Central incisors
10. Lateral incisors
11. Cuspid
12. 1st premolar
13. 2nd premolar
14. 1st molar
15. 2nd molar
16. 3rd molar / wisdom tooth

Lower right:

25. Central incisors
26. Lateral incisors
27. Cuspid
28. 1st premolar
29. 2nd Premolar
30. 1st molar
31. 2nd molar
32. 3rd molar / wisdom tooth

Lower left:

17. 3rd molar / wisdom tooth
18. 2nd molar
19. 1st molar
20. 2nd premolar
21. 1st premolar
22. Cuspid
23. Lateral incisors
24. Central incisors

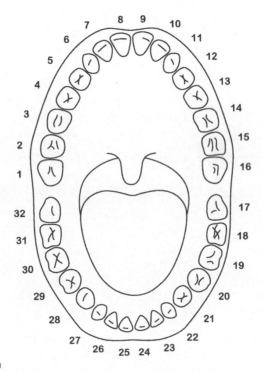

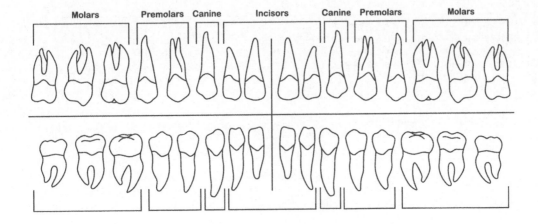

Molars   Premolars   Canine   Incisors   Canine   Premolars   Molars

Dental Anatomy

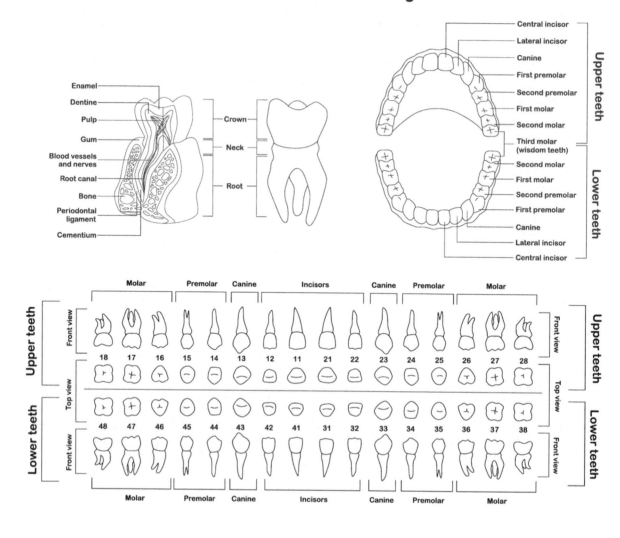

Enamel
Dentine
Pulp
Gum
Blood vessels and nerves
Root canal
Bone
Periodontal ligament
Cementium

Crown
Neck
Root

Central incisor
Lateral incisor
Canine
First premolar
Second premolar
First molar
Second molar
Third molar (wisdom teeth)
Second molar
First molar
Second premolar
First premolar
Canine
Lateral incisor
Central incisor

Upper teeth

Lower teeth

Molar   Premolar   Canine   Incisors   Canine   Premolar   Molar

Upper teeth   Front view

18 17 16 15 14 13 12 11 21 22 23 24 25 26 27 28

Top view

Lower teeth   Top view

48 47 46 45 44 43 42 41 31 32 33 34 35 36 37 38

Front view

Upper teeth   Front view
Top view

Lower teeth   Top view
Front view

Molar   Premolar   Canine   Incisors   Canine   Premolar   Molar

Tooth Anatomy

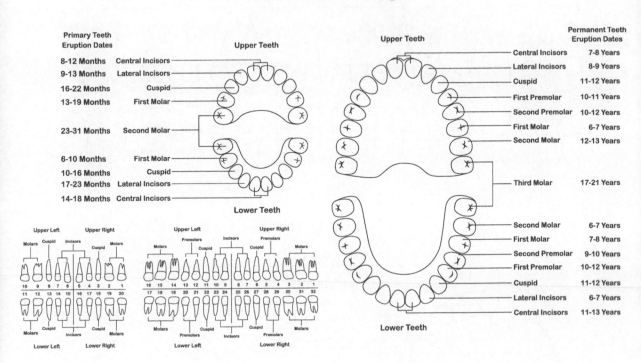

Primary Teeth Eruption Dates

Age	Tooth
8-12 Months	Central Incisors
9-13 Months	Lateral Incisors
16-22 Months	Cuspid
13-19 Months	First Molar
23-31 Months	Second Molar
6-10 Months	First Molar
10-16 Months	Cuspid
17-23 Months	Lateral Incisors
14-18 Months	Central Incisors

Upper Teeth

Lower Teeth

Permanent Teeth Eruption Dates

Tooth	Age
Central Incisors	7-8 Years
Lateral Incisors	8-9 Years
Cuspid	11-12 Years
First Premolar	10-11 Years
Second Premolar	10-12 Years
First Molar	6-7 Years
Second Molar	12-13 Years
Third Molar	17-21 Years
Second Molar	6-7 Years
First Molar	7-8 Years
Second Premolar	9-10 Years
First Premolar	10-12 Years
Cuspid	11-12 Years
Lateral Incisors	6-7 Years
Central Incisors	11-13 Years

Upper Teeth

Lower Teeth

Upper Left   Upper Right
Molars Cuspid Incisors Cuspid Molars
10 9 8 7 6 5 4 3 2 1
11 12 13 14 15 16 17 18 19 20
Molars Cuspid Incisors Cuspid Molars
Lower Left   Lower Right

Upper Left   Upper Right
Molars Premolars Cuspid Incisors Cuspid Premolars Molars
16 15 14 13 12 11 10 9 8 7 6 5 4 3 2 1
17 18 19 20 21 22 23 24 25 26 27 28 29 30 31 32
Molars Premolars Cuspid Incisors Cuspid Premolars Molars
Lower Left   Lower Right

Human Dental Anatomy

Upper teeth

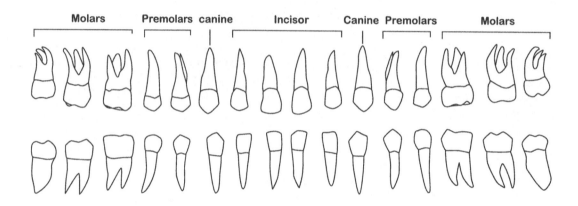

Molars Premolars canine Incisor Canine Premolars Molars

Lower teeth

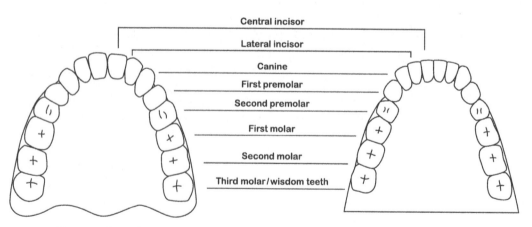

Central incisor
Lateral incisor
Canine
First premolar
Second premolar
First molar
Second molar
Third molar/wisdom teeth

Upper teeth   Lower teeth

Teeth Nembers

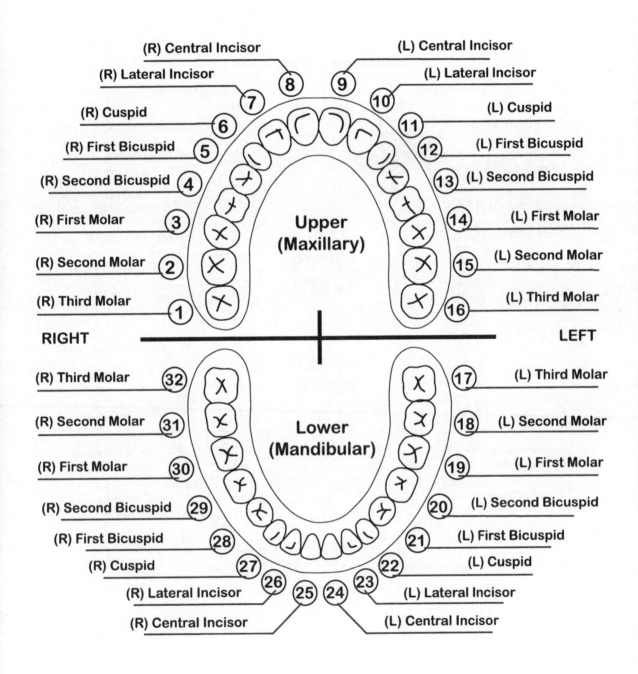

(R) Central Incisor — 8
(L) Central Incisor — 9
(R) Lateral Incisor — 7
(L) Lateral Incisor — 10
(R) Cuspid — 6
(L) Cuspid — 11
(R) First Bicuspid — 5
(L) First Bicuspid — 12
(R) Second Bicuspid — 4
(L) Second Bicuspid — 13
(R) First Molar — 3
(L) First Molar — 14
(R) Second Molar — 2
(L) Second Molar — 15
(R) Third Molar — 1
(L) Third Molar — 16

Upper (Maxillary)

RIGHT   LEFT

Lower (Mandibular)

(R) Third Molar — 32
(L) Third Molar — 17
(R) Second Molar — 31
(L) Second Molar — 18
(R) First Molar — 30
(L) First Molar — 19
(R) Second Bicuspid — 29
(L) Second Bicuspid — 20
(R) First Bicuspid — 28
(L) First Bicuspid — 21
(R) Cuspid — 27
(L) Cuspid — 22
(R) Lateral Incisor — 26
(L) Lateral Incisor — 23
(R) Central Incisor — 25
(L) Central Incisor — 24

DENTAL NUMBERING SYSTEMS

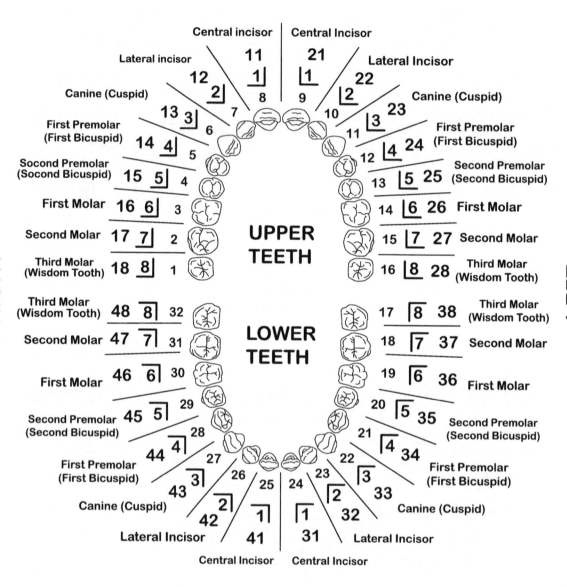

Central incisor 11
Central Incisor 21

Lateral incisor 12
Lateral Incisor 22

Canine (Cuspid) 13
Canine (Cuspid) 23

First Premolar (First Bicuspid) 14
First Premolar (First Bicuspid) 24

Second Premolar (Second Bicuspid) 15
Second Premolar (Second Bicuspid) 25

First Molar 16
First Molar 26

Second Molar 17
Second Molar 27

Third Molar (Wisdom Tooth) 18
Third Molar (Wisdom Tooth) 28

UPPER TEETH

Third Molar (Wisdom Tooth) 48
Third Molar (Wisdom Tooth) 38

Second Molar 47
Second Molar 37

First Molar 46
First Molar 36

Second Premolar (Second Bicuspid) 45
Second Premolar (Second Bicuspid) 35

First Premolar (First Bicuspid) 44
First Premolar (First Bicuspid) 34

Canine (Cuspid) 43
Canine (Cuspid) 33

Lateral Incisor 42
Lateral Incisor 32

Central Incisor 41
Central Incisor 31

LOWER TEETH

RIGHT

LEFT

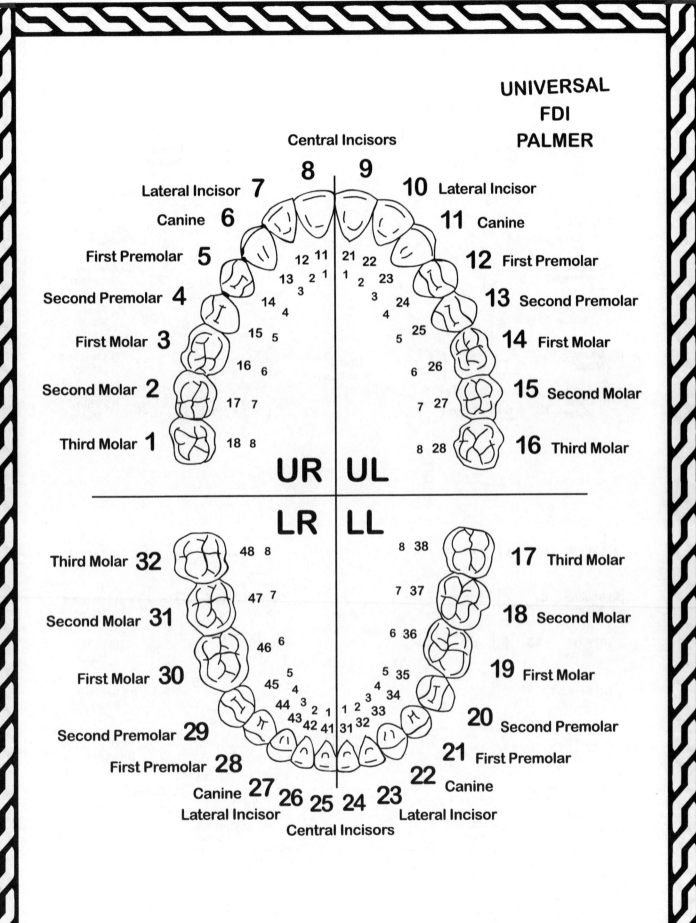

Central Incisors
8 9
Lateral Incisor 7 10 Lateral Incisor
Canine 6 11 Canine
First Premolar 5 12 First Premolar
Second Premolar 4 13 Second Premolar
First Molar 3 14 First Molar
Second Molar 2 15 Second Molar
Third Molar 1 16 Third Molar

12 11   21 22
13 2 1 1 23
14   24
     3   4
15 4   5
   5   25
16 6   6 26
   17 7   7 27
18 8   8 28

UR | UL
LR | LL

Third Molar 32   48 8   8 38   17 Third Molar
47 7   7 37
Second Molar 31   18 Second Molar
46 6   6 36
First Molar 30   19 First Molar
45 5   5 35
44 4   4 34
   3 2 1 1 2 3
43 42 41 31 32 33
Second Premolar 29   20 Second Premolar
First Premolar 28   21 First Premolar
Canine 27 26 25 24 23 22 Canine
Lateral Incisor   Lateral Incisor
Central Incisors

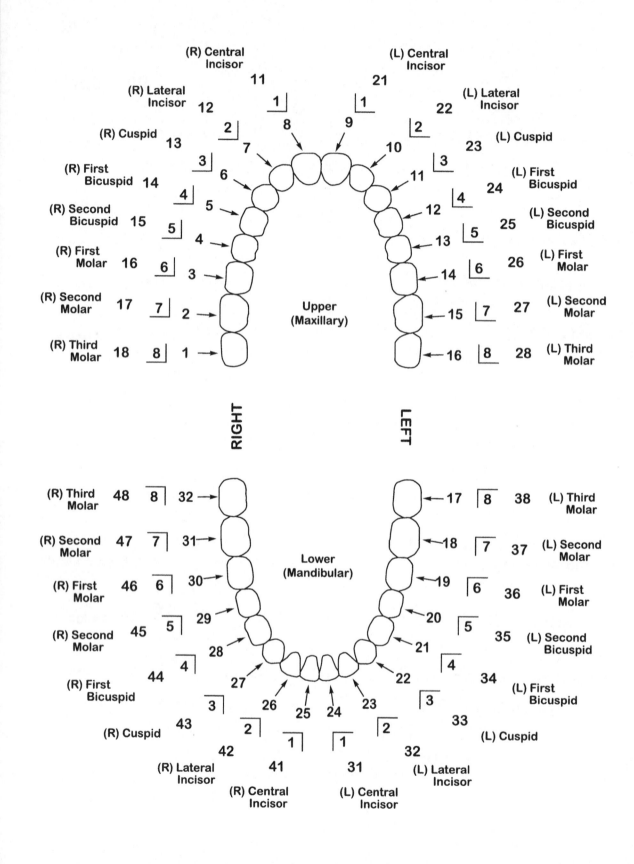

DENTAL NUMBERING SYSTEMS

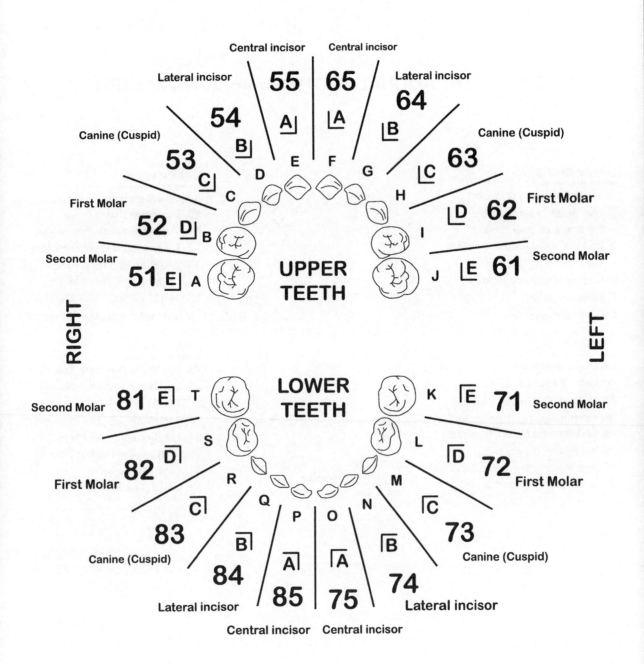

THE INTERNATIONAL TOOTH NUMBERING SYSTEM

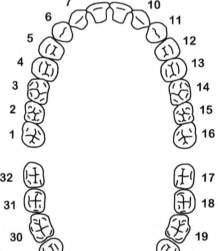

UPPER RIGHT

1. 3rd Molar (wisdom tooth)
2. 2nd Molar (12-year molar)
3. 1st Molar (6-year molar)
4. 2nd Bicuspid (2nd Premolar)
5. 1st Bicuspid (1st Premolar)
6. Cuspid (Canine/Eye tooth)
7. Lateral incisor
8. Central incisor

LOWER RIGHT

25. Central incisor
26. Lateral incisor
27. Cuspid (Canine/Eye tooth)
28. 1st Bicuspid (1st Premolar)
29. 2nd Bicuspid (2nd Premolar)
30. 1st Molar (6-year molar)
31. 2nd Molar (12-year molar)
32. 3rd Molar (Wisdom tooth)

UPPER LEFT

9. Central incisor
10. Lateral incisor
11. Cuspid (Canine/Eye Tooth)
12. 1st Bicuspid (1st Premolar)
13. 2nd Bicuspid (2nd Premolar)
14. 1st Molar (6-Year Molar)
15. 2nd Molar (12-Year Molar)
16. 3rd Molar (Wisdom Tooth)

LOWER LEFT

25. 3rd Molar (Wisdom Tooth)
26. 2nd Molar (12-Year Molar)
27. 1st Molar (6-Year Molar)
28. 2nd Bicuspid (2nd Premolar)
29. 1st Bicuspid (1st Premolar)
30. Cuspid (Canine/Eye Tooth)
31. Lateral incisor
32. Central incisor

Human Dentition

Upper Jaw

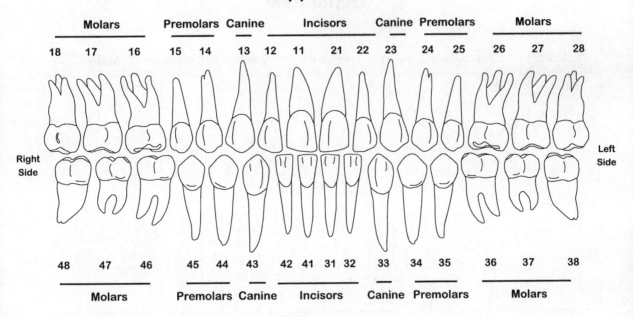

| Molars | Premolars | Canine | Incisors | Canine | Premolars | Molars |

18 17 16   15 14   13   12 11 21 22   23   24 25   26 27 28

Right Side

Left Side

48 47 46   45 44   43   42 41 31 32   33   34 35   36 37 38

| Molars | Premolars | Canine | Incisors | Canine | Premolars | Molars |

Lower Jaw

Permanent Teeth

Tooth Diagram

Upper Jaw

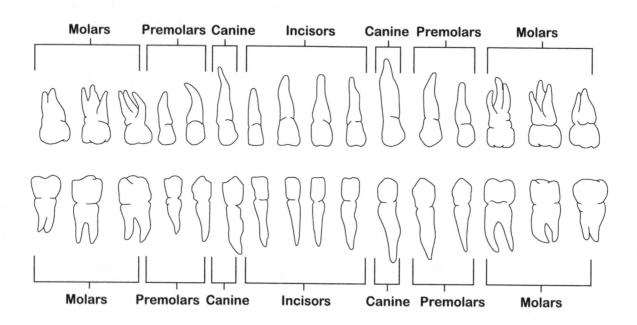

Molars   Premolars   Canine   Incisors   Canine   Premolars   Molars

Molars   Premolars   Canine   Incisors   Canine   Premolars   Molars

Lower Jaw

Upper Jaw Teeth

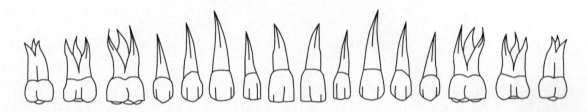

Right Side   **Left Side**

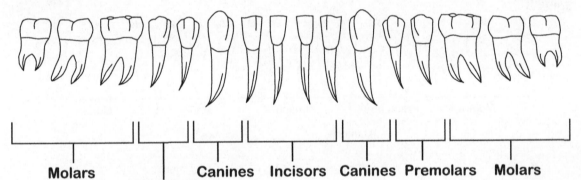

Molars   Canines   Incisors   Canines   Premolars   Molars

Premolars

Lower Jaw Teeth

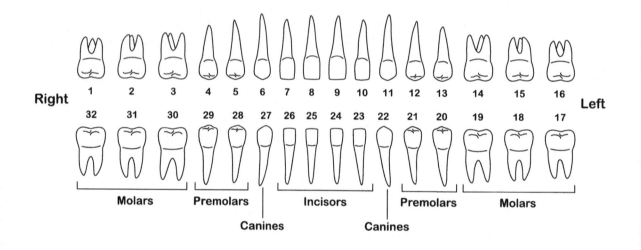

Right   Left

Molars   Premolars   Incisors   Premolars   Molars

Canines   Canines

Molars   Premolars Canine   Incisor   Canine Premolars   Molars

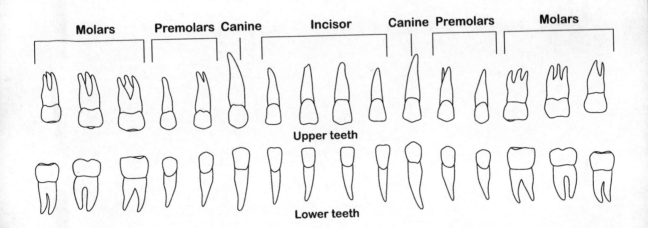

Upper teeth

Lower teeth

Printed in Great Britain
by Amazon

24394716R00040